TA VIDALISTA {TADALAFIL FOR MEN}

Dr. Brandon V. Johnson

Vidalista

Vidalista is suggested for patients who can't accomplish and keep an erection sufficiently able to engage in sexual relations. The dynamic element of Vidalista is tadalafil which is utilized in notable Cialis. Tadalafil gives as long as a day and a half of work contingent upon the patient's age and seriousness of erectile brokenness.

Patients ought to accept Vidalista as recommended by a specialist and try not to take the medication more frequently than 24 hours. Vidalista ought to be taken on a case by case basis, regardless of food.

Moreover, ideally, let's ensure that some other prescriptions you are taking won't communicate with your Vidalista pills. The most risky and, surprisingly, hazardous connections that might occur assuming you take Tadalafil with drugs containing nitrates or nitrites. These are generally heart drugs, and you ought to ensure that you are not taking any.

The dynamic fixing in Vidalista is Tadalafil. This works likewise to Sildenafil, the dynamic fixing in Viagra, by loosening up the veins and accordingly expanding how much blood stream in the private parts. Tadalafil works for much longer, stirring as long as a day and a half so considers greater suddenness and needn't bother with to be taken as frequently. This long activity, has given Tadalafil the moniker "The Weekender".

Vidalista interest has as of late spiked alongside other Indian fake drug, for example, Kamagra among numerous others as men search for less expensive ways of treating ED. Nonetheless, the wellbeing risks of these phony items are notable and announced issues are on the ascent. Fake medications are causing strokes and cardiovascular failures in sound grown-ups who purchase these meds from ill-conceived destinations. The UK government has done whatever it may take to decrease unlawful importation.

To lay it out plainly it's NOT. Vidalista isn't authorized to be legitimately sold in the UK and thusly isn't checked or managed. It's difficult to tell the amount of the dynamic fixing, if any, the pills could contain or on the other hand assuming they contain any destructive added substances that could hurt the body. Added substances and illegal medications were viewed as in a considerable lot of the held onto fake drugs. To put it plainly, regardless of whether you have had great involvement in one cluster of this stuff you can never be certain what will be in the following.

Are There Any Aftereffects?

There are aftereffects to any medication, yet with an unlicensed pill checking every one of the conceivable incidental effects unimaginable. The results of Tadalafil, the dynamic fixing that pills professes to contain, is redness of the eye, cerebral pains, and facial flushing because of the enlargement of veins in pieces of the body other than the penis. As Tadalafil goes on for as long as a day and a half in the body, unsavory secondary effects can keep going this long too. It's likewise conceivable that the pills could contain obscure substances which could cause unsavory aftereffects. There are a few unsafe cooperations of Vidalista that could be risky with the prescription you could currently be on.

For what reason is Men Taking Vidalista?

Erectile brokenness is an extremely normal issue in the UK. It can truly influence the sexual existence of men and lead to additional difficult issues like melancholy. Over portion of men have experienced some type of ineptitude when they arrive at the age of 40 and the pervasiveness is rising consistently. Subsequently numerous men go to purchasing fake drug like Vidalista, and the other famous tablet Kamagra.

There is a typical confusion that taking weakness medication

Increment sexual energy and elevate execution, but this isn't generally the situation. This drug should be endorsed by a specialist as there is generally a potential for serious incidental effects. It can likewise cooperate with different drugs so getting a suggestion from a clinical expert prior to consuming any ED medication is significant.

What are the Lawful Choices from Vidalista perspective?

The dynamic fixing in Vidalista is Tadalafil which is accessible for buy online from trustworthy authorized sources, for example, e-Medical procedure for just £9.50. This prescription is obtained from genuine UK providers, so the quality and intensity are ensured. It will likewise be twofold checked by an authorized UK specialist to guarantee it is entirely ok for you to take.

What is it that I want to be aware prior to taking the Legitimate other options?

Assuming Tadalafil is consumed close by prescription containing

Nitrate it can cause a serious drop in circulatory strain which could demonstrate deadly.

The medication could likewise demonstrate unsafe to anybody experiencing any innate eye illness, liver or kidney issues, or had pelvic medical procedure.

You ought to constantly converse with your PCP or drug specialist prior to ingesting any medications. E-Medical procedure offers a totally free Ask-a-Drug specialist administration which you can use to get additional data from an accomplished drug specialist.

exologists report that it just pauses for a minute to expand the penis up to 6.4 inches, and clinical teachers from Stanford College has exhibited it because of a few clinical trials, which demonstrated that 120 minutes was enough for the corpora cavernosal (huge groups) of the penis to start to develop. Along these lines, the penis fills in size and width, and the erections last longer, and that implies you could fulfill your accomplice up to multiple times in succession.

Teacher of the Stanford College made a speedy and 100 percent regular recipe to expand the size of the penis, and the whole logical world, from sexologists to specialists and scholastics, affirmed that this significant revelation will end an issue that is dishonorable for great many men. Furthermore, this revelation is upheld by free tests and clinical and lab preliminaries, among others.

How compelling are Vidalista tablets?

Because of the unlicensed and unregulated nature of Vidalista, the adequacy of the treatment could be a lot of lower contrasted with clinically demonstrated and tried Tadalafil.

Vidalista comes in numerous qualities:

- ✓ Vidalista 20mg
- ✓ Vidalista 40mg
- ✓ Vidalista 60mg
- ✓ Vidalista 80mg

It is essential to take note of that taking dosages of Tadalafil above 20mg can be destructive to wellbeing and isn't authorized by UK medical services suppliers

Is Vidalista safe?

Vidalista tablets are not directed, as they are not authorized to be legitimately sold in the UK. In this manner, the dynamic fixing, as well as different fixings found in Vidalista tablets, could contain obscure added substances that could be risky to your wellbeing. Moreover, the guaranteed measure of the dynamic fixing can vary from the genuine dose, possibly prompting unfortunate outcomes or intensified secondary effects.

Men with erectile brokenness (ED) may profit from the physician endorsed drug Vidalista Dark 80 mg, which is just open with a specialist's medicine. Tadalafil, the essential part, is a phosphodiesterase type 5 (PDE5) inhibitor. PDE5 inhibitors work by expanding blood stream to the penis to work on erectile capability and sexual execution.

This is the effect of tadalafil. Vidalista Dark 80 mg is ordinarily protected and powerful when taken as coordinated; in any case, there are sure precautionary measures you ought to take to guarantee that you are involving this medicine in a manner that is both protected and compelling for you. We'll turn out a portion of the safety measures you ought to take in the event that you want to eat 80 mg of Vidalista Dark in the accompanying passages.

Vidalista Dark 80 mg is a physician recommended drug that ought to just be utilized under the oversight of a clinical master. Prior to taking Vidalista Dark 80 mg, visit your primary care physician to guarantee that it is the appropriate medicine for you.

To lay out whether Vidalista Dark 80 mg is ok for you, your PCP will audit your clinical history, meds, and any hidden ailments. This is particularly basic in the event that you are taking tadalafil-communicating medications like nitrates, alpha-blockers, or circulatory strain drugs.

You should follow the dosing bearings given by your doctor while taking Vidalista Dark 80 mg. The person will let you know the amount to take each time. The suggested measurements are one pill day to day, required ideally thirty minutes before sexual action.

There is no necessity that the drug be taken with food, despite the fact that it is suggested that high-fat feasts be stayed away from in light of the fact that they can lessen the viability of the medicine. In the event that the measurements are expanded past what is proposed, there is a bigger potential of encountering undesirable impacts. Similarly as with any medicine, quite possibly Vidalista Dark 80 mg could cause a few unwanted incidental effects.

Normal secondary effects incorporate migraines, flushing of the cheeks, nasal clog, irritated stomach, and back torment.

These adverse consequences are generally gentle and disappear all alone. Nonetheless, in the event that you experience serious or tireless secondary effects, you ought to contact your primary care physician at the earliest opportunity. Intriguing however serious secondary effects incorporate unexpected vision misfortune, hearing misfortune, and priapism (a horrendously extended erection).

Liquor and Sporting Medications

Try not to polish off any cocktails or sporting medications assuming that you anticipate taking Vidalista Dark 80mg. Conceivable curing won't fill in too or that you'll make more horrendous side impacts assuming you drink liquor or utilize sporting medications.

They may likewise diminish your capacity to use wise judgment, improving the probability of committing errors that could prompt injury.

Nitrates and Alpha-Blockers

You shouldn't accept Vidalista Dark 80 mg assuming you are as of now under therapy for an ailment that expects you to take nitrates or alpha-blockers. Nitrates and alpha-blockers are the two classes of medications that are utilized to treat different ailments, including chest uneasiness, hypertension, and a broadened prostate. Prior to starting Vidalista Dark 80 mg treatment, you should examine the medications you are all right now taking with your essential consideration doctor. This incorporates non-prescription medications, physician recommended meds, nutrients, home grown enhancements, and dietary enhancements.

There is plausible that taking tadalafil with specific different meds could bring about an expanded gamble of unfavorable impacts or a lessened advantage from taking the medicine.

Medical issue

You might have to utilize Vidalista Dark 80 mg with additional watchfulness in the event that you as of now have a previous clinical issue. On the off chance that you have a background marked by conditions like coronary illness, stroke, or low circulatory strain, for example, you might be at a higher gamble of encountering unfriendly outcomes. Your primary care physician might have to change the dose of the medication assuming that you have a condition that influences either your liver or your kidneys. On the off chance that you have a background marked by vision or hearing hardships, you ought to examine this with your PCP prior to utilizing Vidalista Dark 80 mg. Moreover, on the off chance that you have a background marked by vision issues, you ought to examine this with your primary care physician.

Fake phosphodiesterase-5 inhibitors (PDE-5i) are a rising issue. Currently in far and wide use, the market for PDE-5i is consistently developing as the populace ages. Forgers are exploiting this developing business sector by creating illegal and fake PDE-5i items. Many variables are adding to the quick development of the illegal market, like the okay of arraignment, possibly high monetary prize, and simplicity of dispersion through Web drug stores. Customers of unlawful PDE-5i frequently don't understand they are utilizing fake items and setting themselves at a superfluous wellbeing risk. Others look to sidestep the authentic medical services framework due to one or the other humiliation of the hidden condition or longing for less expensive other options. Be that as it may, taking unlawful PDE-5i may hurt customers straightforwardly, as numerous illegal items contain hindering pollutants and off base measures of the dynamic fixing without the suitable admonitions. Bypassing the genuine medical services framework additionally jeopardizes customers in a roundabout way, as erectile brokenness (ED) is frequently connected with other clinical comorbidities that patients ought to be evaluated for. Besides, PDE-5i can have possibly perilous connections with different drugs that are seldom cautioned against with fake PDE-5i. This correspondence surveys the writing in regards to fake PDE-5i, and sums up both the degree and risks of the illegal PDE-5i market.

The fake medication market is an indistinct and continually developing substance that has become progressively challenging to characterize and evaluate. In 2009, the World Wellbeing Association (WHO) characterized a "fake medication" as one "which is purposely and deceitfully mislabeled concerning personality or potentially source." In any case, numerous in the association have questioned this meaning of fake medication, and there has all the earmarks of being no generally settled upon definition among part conditions of the WHO. Forging can apply to both marked and conventional items. This can incorporate items with true blue fixings, yet with inadequate or exorbitant amounts, items with some unacceptable fixings, or items with tricky bundling. At present, the WHO is utilizing the expression "Unacceptable, Misleading, Dishonestly marked, Misrepresented, and Fake (SSFFC)" for clinical items until another definition is settled upon. For the reasons for this paper, the expression "fake" will be utilized to incorporate all types of SSFFC meds.

No matter what the definition, drug falsifying has turned into a worldwide issue. Notwithstanding the protected innovation privileges that forger's abuse, the items they make can put purchasers in harm's way. Genuine drugs should pass energetic principles and go through enormous, randomized preliminaries prior to being officially supported for people in general. Then, all endorsed meds are made under vigorously checked conditions. Fake meds sidestep this large number of protections

The enormous market for fake drugs isn't similarly appropriated in size or class of prescriptions around the world. It is biggest in poor and agricultural nations, with the size of the market being contrarily corresponding to how much guideline. The extent of misrepresented drugs goes from 1% in industrialized nations that have a very much directed and controlled drug market to as high as 60% in a few non-industrial nations. Nonetheless, even in these all around managed nations, the market for fake PDE-5i has developed. All around the world, anti-microbials contain the biggest class of fake drugs, yet in Europe, PDE-5i is the most normally forged meds. Truth is told, for PDE-5i, the unlawful market in industrialized nation's moves toward the size of that in agricultural nations. Somewhere in the range of 2004 and 2008, 35.8 million fake sildenafil tablets were held onto in Europe, which is multiple times more noteworthy than how much any remaining duplicated Pfizer items consolidated. Two separate examinations in Europe assessed that 0.6 to 2.5 million men are being presented to illegal sildenafil contrasted with around

2.5 million clients of legitimate sildenafil. Be that as it may, the genuine extent of unlawful PDE-5i use is hard to gauge. In one review endeavoring to assess unlawful sildenafil use, convergences of sildenafil and sildenafil metabolites were estimated in sewage

Treatment focuses in the Netherlands. The all out sewage load was back determined to appraise absolute sildenafil utilization, and it was viewed that as more prominent than 60% of recognized sildenafil was not represented by lawful solutions.

What's more, fake PDE-5i frequently contains foreign substances. These are utilized either as building specialists to bring down creation costs or to emulate the appearance and actual characteristics of the certifiable item. In those examples held onto in the Unified Realm, Italy, and Indonesia, there were pollutants like gypsum, non-sanitized powder, amphetamine, business grade paints, paracetamol, and metronidazole. These non-drug fixings can have poison levels of their own. Non-announced drugs can have drug cooperations and secondary effects, for example, gastrointestinal side effects and queasiness while joining metronidazole and liquor. Forgers don't proclaim these fixings or alerts of conceivable harmful collaborations on their bundling.

Besides, the assembling states of forgers can't match the sterile handling states of authentic drugs. In an examination of microbial heaps of different unlawful ED drugs, 23% were debased with in excess of 103 province framing units (CFU), and 69% had raised levels thought about inside adequate cutoff points. Not a solitary CFU was recognized in any of the supported PDE-5i got lawfully (29) (Figure 1). These outcomes are to be expected, while thinking about the severe guidelines and assessments that real drug makers should pass, contrasted and the unsterile conditions in which forgers might work. Numerous labs of forgers are presented to the outdoors and use unsterile water that wouldn't alright for drink. Pollution with either debasements or microbes presents dangers to customers of fake PDE-5i.

Fake PDE-5i posture numerous — perhaps serious — dangers to patients. As the populace ages, and the market for PDE-5i develop, so does the illegal market for PDE-5i. Fake PDE-5i has turned into an overall issue that contains an enormous level of PDE-5i use in both creating and advanced nations. Patients humiliated by their condition or looking for more affordable choices to genuine drugs have powered the market, and the development of Web drugs have made fake drugs simple to acquire. In any case, ED is an ailment that should be treated thusly. By bypassing the authentic medical care framework, clients of fake PDE-5i detour evaluating for simultaneous clinical comorbidities, as well as legitimate schooling and admonitions of PDE-5i use. Moreover, fake PDE-5i frequently contains ill-advised dosing and impurities that might put patients at direct gamble. Many "regular enhancements" contain unlawful PDE-5i, exposing clients to similar dangers with even less advance notice. Doctors who treat ED ought to caution patients against buying PDE-5i through elective means, particularly the Web. The utilization of dietary enhancements for treatment of ED ought to be evaluated for and given due insurances.

Mounting proof shows that erectile brokenness drugs (EDMs) have become progressively utilized as a sexual improvement help among men without a clinical sign. Sporting EDM use has been related with expanded sexual gamble ways of behaving, an expanded gamble for STIs, including episode HIV disease, and high paces of accompanying unlawful medication use. The point of the current review was to explore the attributes and related risk factors for sporting EDM use among youthful, solid, undergrad men. A cross-sectional example of 1,944 men was enrolled from 497 undergrad organizations inside the Joins States between January 2006 and May 2007. The review surveyed examples of EDM use, as well as segment, substance use, and sexual conduct qualities. Four percent of members had casually involved an EDM eventually in their lives, with 1.4% revealing current use. Most of sporting EDM clients detailed blending EDMs in with illegal medications and especially during hazardous sexual ways of behaving. Sporting EDM use was freely connected with expanded age, gay, or sexually unbiased sexual direction, chronic drug use, lifetime number of sex accomplices, and lifetime number of "casual hookups." Sporting EDM clients likewise detailed a 2.5-crease pace of erectile troubles contrasted with nonusers. By and large, sporting utilization of EDMs was related with sexual gamble ways of behaving and substanceEarlier examinations have started to give genuinely necessary information on sporting EDM use; nonetheless, they are not without their constraints. By far most of studies have examined from high-risk populaces, like patients at STI/HIV facilities and anticipation programs, and MSM going to circuit gatherings and clubs, and subsequently little information are accessible with respect to EDM use among hetero men. Second, the greater part of studies has utilized somewhat little comfort tests enrolled from explicit geographic areas, which has restricted the generalizability of these discoveries. Third, concentrates on have not laid out an occasion explicit relationship between EDM use and expanded sexual gamble conduct. In spite of the fact that there has all the earmarks of being a connection between these ways of behaving, more information are required as for the hour of EDM use and the particular type(s) of sexual way of behaving. At long last, a lack of studies has examined EDM use in an undergrad populace. Analyzing EDM use in school matured men might be profitable in light of multiple factors:

(1) People would be moderately youthful and the commonness of clinically huge ED would be very low; and

(2) undergrads report high paces of liquor and illicit drug use, as well as high paces of sexual gamble taking (Cooper, 2002; Gledhill-Hoyt, Lee, Strode, &Wechsler, 2000), ways of behaving which might be related with EDM use.

The current examination was intended to give the main public review directed in the Joins States analyzing EDM use in hetero, sexually open, and gay undergrad men. Our most memorable point was to evaluate the paces of sporting utilization of sildenafil, tadalafil, and vardenafil and investigate graphic attributes connected with their utilization, like recurrence and length of purpose, inspirations for use, source(s) of securing, and corresponding unlawful medication use. Second, we intended to explore related risk factors for sporting EDM use, including segment attributes, as well as sexual way of behaving and substance misuse qualities.

Socioeconomics Members finished an overall socioeconomics poll which included things about age, race/nationality, financial status, scholarly year, geographic home, and sexual direction as evaluated with the Kinsey Sexual Direction scale (Kinsey, Pomeroy, &Martin, 1948).

Erectile Brokenness Prescription Use Men were evaluated with respect to whether they had at any point utilized an oral EDM and, if indeed, the sorts utilized (sildenafil, tadalafil, and vardenafil) and motivation behind use (e.g., to treat ED analyzed by a doctor or for sporting reasons). They likewise detailed whether they presently utilized an EDM and, if indeed, the recurrence of purpose (recent weeks, a half year, and 1 year), and the recurrence by which members regularly knew the dose of the EDM that they were utilizing (1= never, 2=sometimes, 3=about a fraction of the time, 4=most times, 5=always). Inspiration for use was additionally evaluated by having members select every one of the specific intentions that applied to them; reaction choices were: interest, increment erectile inflexibility, decline unmanageable stage, check impacts of medications/liquor that might lessen erection, increment erectile sensation, increment charisma, upgrade confidence, decline execution tension, intrigue/fulfill sexual accomplice, other. Members showed whether they had at any point joined an EDM with sporting medications. Assuming they answered positively, they were approached to provide details regarding the accompanying substances: methamphetamines/amphetamines, MDMA (joy), alkyl nitrites (poppers), ketamine, GHB/GBL (gamma-hydroxybutyric corrosive/γ-butyrolactone), maryjane, cocaine, LSD, mushrooms (psilocybin), heroin, and liquor. Members additionally wrote about the recurrence of attendant medication use (recent weeks, a half year, and year) and whether they accepted that blending EDMs in with illegal medications improved their sexual experience (1=strongly dissent, 2= to some degree deviate, 3=neither concur nor dissent, 4=agree fairly, 5=strongly concur). At last, the essential source by which people obtained EDMs was evaluated, as well as the office by which members procure EDMs (estimated by the accompanying thing, "I have simple admittance to get Viagra, Cialis, or Levitra," scored as 1=strongly deviate, 2= fairly dissent, 3=neither concur nor deviate, 4=agree to some degree, 5=strongly concur).

Erectile Capability Sexual working was surveyed by the Global File of Erectile Capability (IIEF) (Rosen et al., 1997)which is a 15-thing very much approved self-report poll evaluating five spaces of male sexual working: erectile capability (six things), orgasmic capability (two things), sexual longing (two things), intercourse fulfillment (three things), and generally speaking fulfillment (two things). Since a considerable lot of the things on the IIEF are connected with sex inside the beyond about a month, just physically dynamic people finished this poll.

Sexual Conduct Members were found out if they had at any point participated in sex and, if indeed, the age (in years) at which members had encountered their most memorable intercourse, and whether members were right now physically dynamic (participating in intercourse inside the beyond about a month). To assess sexual gamble ways of behaving, members finished things that evaluated their number of sexual accomplices during the beyond 4 weeks, a half year, and 1 year. Reaction choices were 0-1, 2-5, and more than 5. Likewise evaluated were the lifetime number of sexual accomplices (0-10, 11-50, >50), and the quantity of various accomplices with whom members have had sex on one and only one event (casual hookups; 0, 1-5, >5). Kinds of sexual contact (oral, vaginal, butt-centric insertive, butt-centric responsive), as well as whether members utilized condoms or potentially EDMs during these sorts of sexual contact, and members' information on accomplices' HIV status, was additionally analyzed. Reaction choices to these things were estimated as dichotomous (yes/no) reactions. At last, members revealed whether they have at any point gotten a STI during their lifetime. Those detailing yes were approached to demonstrate which type(s) and whether they had at any point participated in unprotected oral-genital sex or unprotected intercourse while showing side effects of a STI.

Male members matured 18 and more seasoned were enrolled by means of online ordered notices as well as through web-based person to person communication destinations (e.g., Live Journal, Xanga) and were approached to partake in a review about "sexual way of behaving and sporting medication use." People were likewise selected through an undergrad brain science subject pool at the College of Texas at Austin. All members were expected to peruse a web-based assent structure prior to accessing the mysterious review. The study didn't utilize treats and didn't gather client IP addresses. No expressly recognizing data was gathered except for the member's scholastic organization wherein he was enlisted, as well as the city and condition of his home. After finish of the 30-min overview, every member was interviewed and given an irregular ID number that filled in as an affirmation that he had finished the study. Members were approached to email these recognizable proof numbers to the essential examiner to such an extent that they could be placed into a month to month wager, whereupon one member was haphazardly chosen every month and sent a check for $50. Members inside the brain science subject pool at the creators' subsidiary college got credit toward their brain science research necessity. The convention was endorsed by the College of Texas at Austin Institutional Survey Board.

Members revealing an erectile capability score of <25 were viewed as encountering erectile brokenness of a clinical sort. This cutoff esteem has been exhibited to have a responsiveness of 0.97 and an explicitness of 0.88 to distinguish people with and without erectile brokenness (Cappelleri, Rosen, Smith, Mishra, and Osterloh, 1999). Sexual direction was sorted based on members' scores on the Kinsey Sexual Direction Scale, by which scores of 0, 1, or 2 indicate hetero sexual personality, scores of 4, 5, or 6 mean gay sexual character, and a score of 3 signifies sexually open sexual personality. Illegal medication use was ordered into the quantity of various medication types (except for EDMs) utilized inside the previous year (0, 1, 2-4, >4), as well as absolute number of medication use events (paying little heed to sedate sort; 0, 1-50, >50). Liquor use was inspected as the normal number of episodes that a member was tanked during the previous week (0, 1-3, >3), as well as the complete number of cocktails consumed during the previous month (0-50, 51-100, >100). Extra investigations involving elective cut focuses for unlawful medication use and liquor use didn't change the outcomes. Current smokers were ordered based on number of cigarettes smoked each day (≥10 cigarettes/day).

Untimely discharge - or PE - is a condition that is more normal than you likely understand. Evaluations of the quantity of men battling with a diagnosable condition range from one of every five to practically 40%, while a lot more men are probably going to report disappointment with their sexual perseverance - regardless of whether they have the condition.

This is probably going to be the consequence of the way that we truly misjudge how much time men last - and the ideal time that sex ought to last itself. As indicated by one review, the typical time a man can have penetrative sex without climaxing is a little more than five minutes. In the interim, anything short of one moment is for the most part considered to comprise PE. On the off chance that the speed of climax is baffling or is joined by other gloomy sentiments, this might be PE as well.

Dissimilar to erectile brokenness, the reasons for PE have not yet been completely explained. While certain clinicians accept it is connected essentially to a mental reason, others have highlighted physiological elements. Also, this vulnerability clearly has its repercussions for treatment: no single viable fix has yet been found.

This reality has made men puzzle over whether Cialis, Viagra, and other erectile brokenness medicines can be utilized to oversee PE. What's more, that is the reason we're thinking about the inquiry today.

Might Cialis at any point Assist You with enduring Longer in Bed?

Tragically, the response to the inquiry may not be the one you were searching for. Cialis isn't authorized as a treatment for untimely discharge - and, therefore, it isn't prompted that you take it for this reason.

This is on the grounds that Cialis has not been demonstrated in that frame of mind to be a dependable treatment for the condition. The initial research facility try into Tadalafil's conceivable treatment of PE, in 2010, didn't show results that were genuinely huge. A later report, in the meantime, found that Cialis protracted the time that men went prior to discharging. Be that as it may, the outcomes here were self-announced, which might think twice about exactness of the information.

The issue with a large part of the examination into the connection among Tadalafil and PE is that it has not been done in a dependable manner. As one audit of studies into the impact of Viagra and Cialis on PE noticed, 13 out of 14 examinations accessible were defective. The last review remembered for the survey tracked down no beneficial outcome of the medication in facilitating the condition.

Accordingly, it can't be dependably said that Cialis can assist with PE. In any case, it can assist you with enduring longer in bed in one significant way. On the off chance that you are not enduring the length of you would like since you can't keep an erection, these erectile brokenness medicines can help - as that is precisely exact thing they are intended for.

What ought to be worried, however, is that men with erectile brokenness appear to be significantly more liable to battle with untimely discharge. As indicated by one review, as numerous as half of men with ED would experience the ill effects of the condition - and Cialis can assist with this as well.

It's felt that the occurrence of the two circumstances might be because of the way that men with ED are bound to race to get done, so as not to lose their erection. Essentially, execution uneasiness connected with ED is remembered to add to the condition as well - as pessimistic sentiments and stress can mediate in and disturb the ordinary cycles of excitement. This can, thus, incite an endless loop wherein further tension forms and the side effects become exacerbated.

In the event that you feel like you are here, Cialis, Viagra, and other ED medicines can help. Men ingesting these medications have been found to have more prominent certainty, diminished tension, and more significant levels of fulfillment coming about because of sex. This could itself at any point help the time that you last prior to discharging - while making you more calm with sex regardless of how long you last.

The two medications take around 30 to an hour to start working and permit patients to accomplish the erection they anticipate. Top fixation in the blood is arrived at following two hours for tadalafil and around one hour for sildenafil. Thusly, we generally propose taking medicine about a little while before sexual movement. The time it takes for the medication to work will fluctuate between patients, so use related knowledge as an aide.

Of note, sildenafil, a conventional Viagra, can be fairly repressed in the wake of eating an enormous feast containing greasy food sources, and this isn't a worry with tadalafil (nonexclusive Cialis). We frequently recommend sildenafil for wedded couples or long haul accomplices with a more unsurprising sexual coexistence. Cialis might be more proper for patients who are dating, as the enormous feasts frequently connected with early dating can make sildenafil be less powerful.

Concerning drug permits an erection to endure longer, the reasonable champ is tadalafil. Sildenafil stays powerful for four to six hours, while tadalafil will empower patients to accomplish erections as long as a day and a half after ingestion, an impact as a rule seen in more youthful patients or lesser levels of ED. In the two cases, the medication doesn't increment want, all things considered taking into consideration a superior erection when the craving is available.

Similarly as with any drug, incidental effects are related with both sildenafil and tadalafil. For the most part, nonetheless, the two medications are all around endured and make not many serious side impacts.

Patients taking sildenafil might encounter cerebral pains, sickness, flushing, stodgy nose, and once in a while, heartburn, or tipsiness. Patients may likewise foster a blue tint to their vision. The greater part of these secondary effects is transient and will vanish in the wake of halting the medication. Loss of vision is a possibly extreme symptom of sildenafil in specific exceptionally uncommon clinical circumstances, and you ought to stop the medication and get clinical assistance right away on the off chance that this happens, as this can, in extremely intriguing cases, lead to long-lasting visual deficiency. Patients with specific eye issues, cardiovascular and metabolic illnesses (elevated cholesterol, hypertension, and type 2 diabetes), and smokers might be at higher gamble.

Patients taking tadalafil have a marginally unique secondary effect profile. Like sildenafil, tadalafil can cause cerebral pains, acid reflux, and nasal clog. Nonetheless, tadalafil can likewise cause interesting side effects like back torment, hack, and upper respiratory plot diseases.

Curiously, while the two medications make side impacts, ongoing investigations have shown that they might lessen the gamble of early demise from coronary illness by up to 25%. This doesn't make them a treatment for coronary illness, nor does it supplant any treatments you may as of now be taking for cardiovascular issues.

The two medications have a somewhat gentle gamble profile. Actually important any secondary effects experienced from tadalafil will ordinarily endure longer on the grounds that the medication stays in the circulatory system essentially longer than sildenafil.

Contrasting Medication Associations

In the event that you've been endorsed ED drug previously, or on the other hand assuming you are searching for a solution now, you will without a doubt be found out if you take nitrates. Nitrates like dynamite can cause an unexpected drop in circulatory strain and even lead to coronary episode or stroke. Patients on dynamite ordinarily have serious cardiovascular issues that make taking ED drug unsafe in any case. Patients taking sporting "poppers," including amyl nitrate, amyl nitrite, and butyl nitrate, shouldn't accept ED prescription. Address your primary care physician or drug specialist about other medication communications to guarantee wellbeing while taking your ED prescriptions.

Dr. Engel likes to analogize erectile brokenness to a thrill ride. Ordinarily, there is a sluggish development toward ED. Notwithstanding, when erectile brokenness starts disrupting sexual action, a descending incline for the most part can't be switched. Erectile brokenness prescriptions assist with further developing blood stream to the penis to some extent briefly. Notwithstanding, the hidden vascular issues related with ED regularly deteriorate with age, and that's just the way it is. Accordingly, in the end, these medications will presently not offer fulfilling erections, so, all in all we want to think about additional medicines, including infusions or penile prostheses (inserts).

The accompanying outcomes relate to just those members revealing sporting EDM use and these are likewise displayed in Table 2. Albeit these people had a mean IIEF erectile capability score that was well inside the nonclinical range (M=26.3;SD= 0.63), roughly 27%of these members had ED according to men revealing unprotected open butt-centric intercourse with an accomplice of serodiscordant or obscure HIV status, 73% detailed that they had simultaneously utilized EDMs. Paces of occasion explicit EDM use for men detailing unprotected penetrative butt-centric intercourse and unprotected vaginal intercourse with an accomplice of serodiscordant or obscure HIV status were 63% and 35%, individually.

Recurrence and broadness of substance use were both freely connected with sporting EDM use. Elucidating information uncovered comparative outcomes, with almost 50% of the example of sporting EDM clients announcing correspondingly blending EDMs in with liquor or potentially illegal substances, the most widely recognized of which were pot, liquor, bliss, methamphetamines, and cocaine. These discoveries were like different examinations analyzing examples of sporting medication and EDM use in young fellows (Chu et al., 2003; Kim et al., 2002; Musacchio et al., 2006). A troubling finding was that a sizable extent (15%) of the example revealed blending alkyl nitrites (poppers) with EDMs, a training which is restoratively contraindicated as it might expand the gamble of possibly deadly cardiovascular entanglements (Ishikura et al., 2000). One more place of concern is that most of men who blended EDMs in with sporting substances did as such during sexual action. EDMs in mix with illegal medications might allow men in modified states to participate in risky sexual ways of behaving, making worry for STI and HIV transmission, as well as undesirable pregnancy.

Men who casually utilized EDMs revealed high paces of unprotected intercourse with people of serodiscordant or obscure HIV status. Albeit these rates differed by sexual movement, they were all high (penetrative butt-centric intercourse=63%, responsive butt-centric intercourse=73%, vaginal intercourse=35%). Studies looking at paces of unprotected butt-centric sex with an accomplice of obscure or contrasting HIV serostatus in men have revealed comparable outcomes. These examinations tracked down an expansion in unprotected butt-centric sex with an accomplice of obscure or serodiscordant HIV status among sildenafil clients, with sporting clients somewhere in the range of two and multiple times as prone to participate in this hazard conduct (Chu et al., 2003; Colfax et al., 2001;

Kim et al., 2002; Sherr, Bolding, Maguire, and Elford, 2000). In any case, it is vital to take note of that, after we controlled for segment, substance use, and sexual way of behaving covariates, these sexual gamble taking ways of behaving were not freely connected with EDM use. Besides, sporting EDM use was not freely connected with negative wellbeing results like STIs (counting HIV disease), as revealed in different examinations (Jackson, 2005; Kim et al., 2002).

In our review, men revealing a gay or sexually open sexual personality were roughly 3 to 3.5 times as prone to report EDM use, contrasted with hetero men. This is in accordance with a review that enrolled men looking for public STI administrations in San Francisco, by which gay and sexually unbiased men were multiple times as prone to report sporting EDM use. Another review evaluating sporting EDM use in the Assembled Realm tracked down comparable outcomes (McCambridge, Mitcheson, Chase, and Winstock, 2006). Also, more seasoned age was related with sporting EDM use. This is as per different examinations announcing expanding EDM rates with expanding age, even in examples of young fellows with somewhat little age ranges (Benotsch et al.,

2006; Chu et al., 2003;Musacchio et al., 2006; Santtila et al., 2007). Sporting EDM clients were likewise more physically unhindered contrasted with nonusers. In particular, men who casually use EDMs revealed essentially larger quantities of lifetime sexual accomplices as well as bigger quantities of casual hookups. As a matter of fact, men revealing in excess of 50 sexes and in excess of 5 one-night were roughly 10 and multiple times as liable to casually utilize EDMs, separately.

A significant highlight note is that the presence of clinically huge self-detailed erectile troubles was autonomously related with EDM use. Albeit the mean IIEF erectile capability score of sporting EDM clients was well inside the nonclinical range, 27% of these men had ED, contrasted with 11% of nonusers. The 2.5-crease pace of ED in sporting EDM clients might be made sense of by ongoing information specifying the connection between nonprescription EDM use and trust in erectile capacities. Santtila et al. (2007) found that youthful sporting EDM clients exhibited altogether less trust in their capacity to acquire and keep up with erections contrasted with nonusers, and the recurrence of EDM use was fundamentally adversely corresponded with erectile certainty. Taking into account that absence of trust in one's capacity to start and hold erections has been distinguished as a significant psychogenic gamble factor for ED (Rosen, Cappelleri, Smith, Lipsky, and Pena, 1999), men who use EDMs casually might be powerless against turning out to be mentally subject to erections that are pharmacologically prompted. This is a significant thought thinking about that the biggest expansion in sildenafil use among monetarily guaranteed grown-ups in the U.S. is among more youthful men matured 18-45 years, who had an expansion being used of 312% from 1998 to 2002 (Delate, Simmons, and Motheral, 2004). That being said, one can't preclude the likelihood that regular substance use (which can freely cause erectile challenges) might be etiologically answerable for the expanded pace of self-announced ED. Tragically, this can't be learned by our information, given the cross-sectional nature of our review plan, as well as the way that we didn't explicitly survey this relationship.

(1) The enrollment of a huge, geologically different example of men;

(2) Evaluating pace of purpose and related risk factors in a moderately okay populace (contrasted with men selected from STI/HIV facilities and MSM enlisted from circuit parties) to constrict misjudgment predispositions;

(3) Enlistment of an enormous extent of hetero men;

(4) Evaluation of purpose of every one of the three FDA-endorsed phosphodiesterase inhibitors;

(5) The utilization of a mysterious study led through the web, in this way diminishing social attractiveness inclination and underreporting;

(6) the foundation of occasion explicit relationship between both EDM use and unlawful medications, and EDM use and sexual gamble conduct, as well as time-delicate information in regards to each of the three of these qualities; and

(7) The utilization if thorough measurable techniques to control for related risk factors like age, and sexual direction, as well as substance misuse and sexual conduct attributes.

A few constraints of this study warrant notice. Because of the cross-sectional nature of this review, we recognize the need to practice alert in making direct relaxed derivations of any sort. The relationship between sporting EDM use and sexual gamble ways of behaving warrants further examination, as planned investigations in various populaces, to lay out transience of EDM utilize going before sexual gamble ways of behaving, as well as an expected causal connection between sporting EDM use and expanded chance of psychogenic ED.

Made in the USA
Las Vegas, NV
28 December 2023

83666101R00026